Your Baby's First Year

Enjoying Your Baby's First Year
With
Baby Sign Language

By Nicole Johnson

Copyright @2017

information is without contract or any type of guarantee assurance.

The trademarks that are used are without any consent, and the publication of the trademark is without permission or backing by the trademark owner. All trademarks and brands within this book are for clarifying purposes only and are the owned by the owners themselves, not affiliated with this document.

Table of Contents

BONUS!

Wouldn't be nice to discover and learn sleep tips for babies in a such way that you would sleep while your angel sleep well. Well now is your chance!

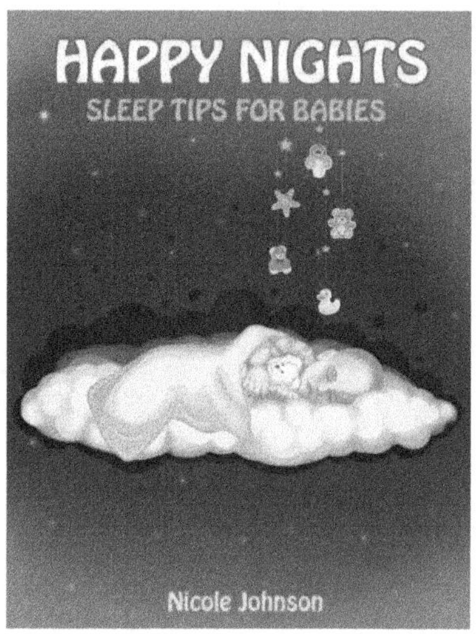

Please check it out   http://bit.ly/2BXvkaZ

Simply as a 'Thank you' for downloading this book, I would like to give you full access to an exclusive that will email you notifications when Amazon's top Kindle Books go on Free Promotion. If you are someone who is interested in saving a ton of money, then simply click the link for FREE access.

Introduction

Your due date is drawing near and you are filled with more emotion than you know how to handle. Your mind is going a hundred miles an hour at all times, and you aren't even sure where to begin to slow it down. There is nothing you want more than to give your child the best start in life possible, but you're worried.

You have heard so much conflicting advice about how you should raise your child through the first year. Some say to only do one thing. Others say to never do that same thing. Some say that you are going to naturally know what to do while others say that you need to take classes before you'll be ready.

You know some of the things you want, but at the same time, you second-guess yourself. How do you know you are doing the right thing? How do you know for sure that you are giving your child everything you could be giving them?

How do you know what they want? And all through all of this, what about you?

When are you going to sleep? When are you going to have some time to yourself? When are you going to get a glimpse of the life that you used to have? There are so many questions swirling around in your mind, how do you know that life is as it should be?

Thankfully, you have come to the right place. In this book, I am going to show you the answer to all of these things and more. You are going to learn what to expect throughout the first year as well as advice on how to make that first year not only bearable but enjoyable.

This book has all the answers you have been looking for, and in it, you are going to discover the key to your baby's first year. Whether this is the first time you are a parent or if you simply want to do things a little differently now than you did before, this is the book for you.

Now, enough of all the chatter – there is going to be plenty of time for that when your baby is down for a nap.

Let's get started.

Part 1: The First Year

Chapter 1:

You're Having a Baby

Let's face it, this past year has gone by in a whirl. You have gone from living your life a certain way to doing a complete turnaround – and most of this has happened to you while you try to keep up with the changes. From the moment you found out you were expecting, all you could think about was this new chapter in your life.

It may have come as a surprise or it may have been something that you have been wanting and working for over the course of months. However, your life made this change, and the fact is that you are now on your way to parenthood, and as the time draws near, you are getting ready to make the leap.

Of course, you have heard your fair share of advice from well-meaning friends and family. People who really want nothing more than to offer you only their best advice and opinions. Although, more often than not, you find that these opinions and tidbits of advice tend to conflict with each other as often as you hear them.

You don't want to hurt anyone's feelings, and you certainly want to be the best parent that you can be, but you know that the closer your due date comes, the more stressed out you feel. You wonder how you are going to take care of your baby, and how you are going to remember everything that they need in order to grow happy and healthy.

You know you would do anything for the happiness of your child, but when it comes to knowing everything there is to know, you feel lost. Not only are there so many things that you need to remember in the care of your child, but there is also a list of things you need to remember to take care of yourself, too.

Parenthood, although it is one of the best things that could ever happen to you, it is also going to be one of the most stressful, especially during the first year. You don't want to spend this year chasing sleep and barely keeping things together as you watch your child go from the infant in your arms to a walking toddler. No, you want this to be one of the happiest, most memorable times of your entire life.

But in order to make that happen, you are going to have to have an idea of what you are doing. You can't just go through the motions, and you certainly can't take all the opposing advice you hear from your friends and family. If this is going to be the best year of your life, you are going to have to make that happen.

You are holding in your hands the secret to turning the coming year into that year you have been dreaming of. Trust me, it's not going to be easy, but it is going to be more than worth it. You are about to step into the best season of your life, and it's one that is going to last the rest of your days.

You'll learn the different stages, you watch as your child grows from the tiny infant you hold in your arms into a beautiful young man or woman, and you will have the pride and joy of being there for them every step of the way. This book is going to show you how to kick off that journey in the best way possible, and you are going to see just how easy it is for you to get through that first year.

Get ready to be the friend who can give advice that actually works. Get ready to be the go-to guru for all their baby needs. Not only are you going to have the answers for your friends, but you are going to be able to watch your own child grow, learn, and love you like you have never been loved before.

This book is going to give you everything you need to get started in the right direction, and you are going to fall in love with the results. You'll sleep better, you'll feel great, and you will watch your baby grow into everything you have ever hoped for them to be – all while, you get to stand next to them every step of the way. This is the best thing that could ever happen to you and it's time to take charge and push it in the right direction.

Get ready for parenthood.

Chapter 2:

The First Month

The first month of your child's life is going to be a roller coaster of emotions. There are going to be so many changes to your baby (and yourself) that you are going to find that things can be completely different on a day to day basis.

You are definitely going to be under the watchful eye of the nurses or the midwife for the first day or two, but once you bring your baby home, you are going to be the one in charge. Yes, this might sound alarming, but if you know what to expect – what is normal and what isn't – then you are going to find that this first month is a lot less scary than what you may have originally anticipated.

Obviously, it all starts at the beginning, and you can't start the first month without the first week – so that is where we, too, will begin our journey.

Week 1

The first week of your baby's life is going to largely consist of them eating, pooping, sleeping, and crying. In the beginning, crying is not only the most effective way of communication, but it is also their only way of communicating. As a parent, you are going to learn what your baby's cries mean, and within a few days, you are going to know the difference between them being hungry and them crying because they need to have their diaper changed.

At the same time, you are going to see changes in their skin. There might be white bumps or red blotches or red bumps – all of this is entirely normal, and it is your job to leave them alone. It all goes away on its own, and the more you can refrain from touching it or doing anything to it, the easier it is going to be. At the same time, you are going to experience a variety of changes in your own body.

During this first week, you are going to bleed from your breast and it will become extremely tender – especially if you are breastfeeding. During this time, having the right fitting bra is going to make all the difference in how you feel as you get through your day, although you can anticipate being really tired during this week.

Week 2

There are two huge changes you can expect that will happen in the second week of your child's life. The first of these two is the growth spurt, as you are going to see a noticeable difference in how your child's clothes fit during this time. This is the time when you are going to be able to start introducing other clothes from your baby's closet as well as begin thinking about getting rid of some of the first clothes you were using.

Week 2 is also when the dread Colic sets in. It is unknown what causes Colic in a newborn child, but up to 20% of babies experience this. Colic is when your baby cries – and cries – and cries nonstop. There doesn't appear to be any reason for this and it doesn't seem to matter how hard you try to soothe them, they continue with their wails, sometimes for hours.

Some suspect that the reason for this is indigestion, as a result of a baby's immature digestive system or something in the environment that is irritating to your baby, although it is impossible to say for sure what is going on. When you are dealing with a colicky baby, keep in mind that patience is key – be rest assured that your child is going to grow out of this stage sooner rather than later.

Just keep your chin up and get ready to move on into the next stage of your baby's life.

Week 3

You can expect new changes in the third week. By now, you are going to know for sure what cries mean what for your child, but you are also going to find that your baby is a lot more in touch with expressing these things to you. At the same time, you can expect your baby to make a lot more noise in his diaper as his digestive system comes into high gear.

At the same time, you are going to be ready for the next stage in your baby's development – start introducing more complex shapes instead of just the basic shapes, and consider using a pacifier during the day instead of just a bottle or breastfeeding.

This is also the stage in which your child is going to be better prepared for the outside world – get ready to start taking outings, although do keep in mind that the world is full of germs and you need to ensure that your baby stays healthy, especially if this time occurs during the cold and flu season.

For you, the mom, this is the week when you may want to begin considering doing some light exercises and massages on your stomach, helping your body return to the state it was in before the hormones took over. Of course, this is going to be somewhat painful at first, but the more time passes and the more you stick with it, the easier it's going to get and the better you are going to feel.

This is a great time to start talking to your mom, and other women you know who have had children, and see what they did that worked for them – you are going to want plenty of advice during this time.

Week 4

By week 4, your baby is going to communicate with you regularly. You'll hear gurgles and coos on a regular basis, and by now, sneezing and hiccups have become part of the regular routine. You are now going to be an old pro at the different cries your baby makes, as well as what their communication style is.

Even at this young age, your child has a personality that is unique to them, and they are going to interact with you accordingly. It is now that you are going to want to start personally strengthening your own body once more – especially below your belt.

You may now be familiar with the different sounds that are coming from down there, and odds are you are going to be doing things that will get rid of them. One of the best ways to do this is to strengthen the floor of your pelvis through the exercise called.

Kegels are the exercise that you do when you strengthen your pelvic floor – squeeze the base of your pelvis and release, then repeat this several times over. The more you do this, the stronger your pelvic floor is going to get, and the less you are going to be hearing those funny sounds coming from inside your underwear.

By now, you are going to be surprised at how much of a pro you are when it comes to childcare – it's amazing how fast that happens.

This means you are going to:

1. Cope. The first month is going to be a month of surprises, and it is going to be the month that you adjust from life as you knew it to a completely new way of doing things. You are going to have to adjust everything to learn how you are going to live your life now – as well as figure out the sacrifices you need to make.

2. You are going to take a step back and re-evaluate. You had expectations and things that you thought were going to be one way, but now that your little joy has arrived, you are going to need to think of things in an entirely new light. Don't rush things.

3. Begin preparing yourself for what lies ahead. You, your spouse, and your baby will experience a major change in the first month. You are going to be responsible for taking care of your child, but at the same time, there is a future that is coming, and you are going to have to be prepared for that as well.

4. Don't rush things. Many times, new parents think that they need to rush. No – your baby is now here, you are responsible for taking care of them, so just let things happen as they do and be prepared for what comes next.

Chapter 3:

What's Next: Months 2 – 4

There are going to be a lot of changes in your baby from month 2 to 4, especially in the 3rd month. It is during this time that your baby is going to go from someone who lies on the bed or on the floor all the time to being able to look toward your voice when you speak to her.

Since your baby is going to be showing more interest in you when you speak to him, set aside a couple hours during the day to turn off the radio and television so your baby can interact with you without the distraction of other noises. This is going to make it easier for you to interact and bond with your child, as well as help them hear words and communicate back with you.

It is also during this time you are going to find that your baby is able to sit up straighter – that they are able to hold their head up by themselves while they are sitting, and that they are even able to stand with your help. They are going to be far more wiggly during this time, kicking with a lot more force and able to move themselves about.

Of course, your top priority is going to be safety throughout all your child's life, but the more mobile your baby becomes, the more care you are going to have to take to ensure they are safe.

Your baby could potentially wiggle off the bed or chair, or even out of your lap if you aren't careful. Make sure you have your hands on your baby at all times when you are holding them, and that you are still providing them with as much security and support like before. Of course, you are going to be far more comfortable taking care of your baby during this time than you were when you first began, but you can't let your guard down next.

It is also during this time that you are going to be encouraging your baby to interact with you. We are going to talk more about baby sign language later, but in addition to that, you can mimic the noises your baby makes when he talks to you.

The 2 to 4 month time span is when your baby is going to become a lot more aware of and in control of their motor skills – meaning you are going to see them open and close their hands, coordinate their hand movements with their eyes, and show an interest in the different items that are around them.

Again, you are going to keep safety as the top priority with your child. The more forceful kicks and expanded movement your child does, the more likely your child could pull something down on top of themselves, or they could accidentally kick something over that they shouldn't.

Some babies will begin to mimic noises they hear at this time – you might hear your baby call you mama or say dada – or you might hear them mimic some of the other simple sounds around your house.

You can work with your baby on certain noises or you can continue to speak to them as you always have – either way, you are going to see specific development in your child during this time, and you are going to find that they show excitement in the things that are going on around them.

Interaction with your child is important during this time. Make sure you are engaging your child in a variety of activities, and that you are working with them to continue with their development each passing day. Your child is going to naturally start picking up on things in the world around them, but you can enhance this if you work with your child and do what you can to ensure they are learning more each day.

You will be taking your child to the doctor for regular visits during this time – and this is going to give you the chance to talk to your doctor and learn what you can do to help your child develop further. This is going to be a process for both you and your child – yes, you are going to see your child doing most of the changing, but during this time, you are going to be developing as a parent as well.

Enjoy the time you spend together, and work together to reach the next step. It is certainly all going to be coming naturally, but at the same time, you are going to be entering each stage together. It is a time of change and love for both of you.

1. **What this means:** It is around month 2 that you are going to start introducing sleep cycles. This is something that many parents struggle with, but it is crucial that if you want to have a chance of sleeping through the night yourself, prepare your child's room for sleeping and success, then begin with the sleeping pattern.

2. Put your child on a routine and make sure you stick to this routine no matter what. If there is a company in the house, you are still going to stick to the routine. If you are traveling, you are going to stick to the routine as much as possible. If something comes up and you can't stick to the routine as much as you would like, you are going to have to adjust to still keep things as

normal as you can while getting through whatever it was that came up.

3. Prepare your baby for bed the same way every night. This can be with a story, a bath, singing, or just winding down together. Your baby is going to get used to the cycle of things and when you do the same thing every night right before bed, your child is going to adjust to this and start to relax when the routine starts.

4. Don't be afraid to feed your baby before bed. Although there are some that say you shouldn't as this is going to keep your child up in the night, it has actually been shown that babies sleep just fine with a full stomach. In fact, this is going to lessen your child waking up in the night hungry and needing you.

5. Be patient with your child. You can train them to sleep through the night, but this is something that does take a bit of time. If you are consistent and start early in your child's life, you are going to find that they are going to take to it a lot better than if you try when they are older. Start young.

6. As your child gets older, don't be afraid to let them cry for a short period of time before you rush to their aid. With a younger baby, you are going to go into the room when they need you, but many times, parents teach their babies that if they wish to be held, all they need to do is fuss and they are going to get it.

   This tends to make it harder to teach your child to sleep through the night as your baby is going to expect you to come running in every time they make a sound. If you allow your baby to cry – for no more than ten minutes, but up to ten minutes – you are going to teach them that they are able to go back to sleep themselves and that they don't need you to come in and hold them every time they wake.

Getting your child to sleep through the night is something many parents hope for with their kids, but it is one thing that many find difficult to teach. Though it can be difficult – especially since no parent wants to hear their child cry – it is something that can be done through loving consistency. The more you teach your child to fall asleep on their own, the more likely they are to stay asleep when they fuss in the night.

Chapter 4:

Halfway There: Six Months In

Once you reach six months, you have reached the halfway point for your child's first year. It has been a roller coaster up to this point, and you have seen a lot of changes take place in your child's life. By now, however, you wouldn't believe the changes that have taken place, the ones that are currently happening, and how you are going to keep up with them.

When it comes to the six month mark, there are a lot of different things that all fall into the category of normal. Your baby may have a tooth at this point, some babies have more than one. At the same time, if your baby doesn't yet have a tooth, it is also normal, and you can expect those to start showing up at any time.

By now, your baby is going to be able to sit up alone, and you will find that they reach for anything they can get their hands on and immediately put whatever it is directly into their mouths. At this time, it is paramount to know that there is no limit to the things your baby will put in his mouth, and if he/she can get his hands on it, in it goes, so you have to supervise to make sure there is nothing dangerous about it.

Though many parents wonder if it is a good idea to allow their child to put anything in their mouth, keep in mind that this is how your baby is going to get used to the world around them. As infants, our brains are designed to connect and explore the world through the things that are put in our mouths.

It might seem strange to an adult, but for a child, this is one of the best ways they can learn – so make sure you have a supply of baby toys on hand that are safe for your child to use, and that you wash these toys frequently to ensure that your baby is not putting anything that is full of germs directly into their mouth, either.

It is close to the six month mark that your baby is going to start becoming mobile. You might find that your baby has rolled over from front to back or vice versa, or that your baby lifts himself up on all fours and rocks back and forth.

Your baby has been watching you and what you're doing all this time, and around the six month mark, they are going to begin mimicking that as well. If they aren't already crawling, you are going to see your baby do this rocking motion as they prepare for the movement themselves. Another common thing during this time is for your baby to rock backwards – and only backwards.

Many babies start their crawling career by backing themselves right into a corner – something that is not only adorable but is also preparing them for crawling normally in the near future. Keep in mind that crawling is not the only thing you can do that will help your baby, too. It is during this time that your baby is going to enjoy standing with your help and dancing around while standing on a hard surface. Again, bear in mind that your baby is going to need your complete support during this time as there is no way for them to hold themselves up.

During this time, you are going to shift your role from doing everything for your child to guiding your child as they begin to learn and take care of themselves. Of course, you are going to be the one who still provides everything – and you will be for months to come – but you are going to see your baby start on solid foods, be able to feed themselves with certain solid foods, and also be able to do more things independently.

If you have been working with your child on their sign language, you will find that at this point, they are fluent with being able to communicate with you through signs, not to mention at this point, their vocabulary is going to be a lot more extensive than it has been. You'll be hearing more and more words clearly and your child will pick up on learning new words a lot faster – though you still won't be hearing them say any extensive sentence at this point.

The six month point is when your child is going to be a wonderful mix of mobile and fearless. They are going to want to engage with the world around them more than ever before, but at this point, you are going to have to be their eyes, ears and shield against everything they can get their hands on. They will have the ability to get into things that they haven't been able to before, and they are not only going to be demanding a lot more of your attention, but they are also going to be needing it as well.

You are going to have to put everything that you normally do on hold once again and spend most of your time chasing around your child, making sure things are picked up and out of their way, all the while taking care of them and helping them explore the world around them.

What this stage means for you:

As the parent, you are the one who knows what is safe and what isn't for your child. You are going to spend this time taking care of them while still allowing them to explore the world and learn new things on their own.

This means you are going to:

1. Make sure the floor and surrounding areas your baby is playing in are completely free of all hazards and danger of all kinds. You will need to be the source of protection for your baby, and you are going to have to make sure they are safe and secure no matter where they are in your house.

2. You are going to be their support – as your child strengthens their muscles, you are going to be the one who helps keep them upright and prevents them from falling over as they learn how to use their legs.

3. You will be working with your child to develop a vocabulary that is both physical and spoken. By now, you are both going to be able to communicate well through sign language and other sources.

4. You are going to take the time with your child to daily interact with them on a one-on-one basis without the distractions of anything electronic. This is going to give your child the chance to converse with you without having the distractions of other things around them.

5. You will be responsible for helping your child start on solid foods. They are going to be able to feed themselves in some ways, and you are going to be there to help them in others.

Chapter 5

Baby Einstein: Your Little Genius

At six months of age, a lot would've changed. The months that follow this to the first year are months that are going to be spent learning a variety of new things, and it is a time when you can greatly aid in your child's developmental process.

Your baby will learn a lot of things naturally, but this is a time when you can take a more hands-on approach to teaching things that your child needs to learn. This ranges from their vocabulary to motor skills and virtually everything in between.

You can use books and teaching DVDs and TV programs to do this, as well as your own experience. Have fun teaching your child how to do new things and stand by them as they learn and grow. It is also during this time that your baby is going to advance in the things that they already know how to do.

The kinds of solid foods your baby can have will increase, your baby's sleeping patterns will be a lot more solid, and you'll find that you are changing your baby's diaper at regular times – and less frequent times – than ever before.

1. **What this means:** This is still a time of developmental growth and change for your baby, but it doesn't mean that you are going to take a step back by any means. Your baby is going to need you through

each and every stage, and you are going to see changes throughout.

2. You are going to take your baby to regular doctor's appointments all throughout this time, and it is there that you are going to hear how your child is doing and what you can do to help them develop further. At the same time, your doctor can give you feedback on your baby's growth as well as advice on nutrition and other basic needs.

3. You are going to see your baby go from crawling to walking during these months, as well as learning how to do things, such as opening drawers, doors, navigating stairs, and other things that are similar to this.

4. You can engage with your child in a variety of ways during this time, and many of those things are going to come through your hands-on approach. Talk to your doctor about ways you can increase this and things you can do that will help your child.

5. Be patient and enjoy this time. You are going to see many wonderful changes in your baby, and you are going to be there for them through it all. It's nothing you can rush, but it's certainly something that you can enjoy every step of the way. In the chapters to come, I am going to show you how you can make the most of this time for yourself – growing your relationship with your partner, finding time for yourself, and getting that coveted sleep you need.

Hang on, you are coming up on your child's first year.

Chapter 6

Your One Year Old

At one year of age, your baby is going to seem like a whole new child compared to what you were used to facing over the past year. At first, the changes are going to be deliberate and swift, but with time, they are going to grow into subtle changes that will creep up on you when you least expect it.

Cue the first year.

You have been by your child's side all through the past year, standing by them as they went from being a newborn to the blossoming toddler you see before you. From the moment you brought your child home until now, you have been watching him/her grow and change with the times. And you have been rooting him along every step of the way.

But what's next? What lies in the year to come?

Compared to the first few weeks of your child's life, it might seem like smooth sailing from here on out, but that's not entirely true. In fact, while your job as a parent has gotten easier in some senses of the word, there are certain things that you are now going to have to watch out for and be aware of that are going to play major roles in your child's life.

The first thing you need to be aware of is that your baby is going to be far more mobile this year and it's only going to get harder for you to keep an eye on him.

That's right, if your baby isn't walking already, you are fast approaching the time in your baby's life when he is going to be. Now, while this is both scary and exciting, there are a few things that you are going to need to do to ensure it is a safe and smooth transition.

For starters, rearrange your home so the furniture is placed around the room, making it easy for your child to use it as support as he walks from one room to the other. At the same time, you are going to have to let your baby do more things on his own during this time – a transition that can be difficult for some parents to understand.

Your baby needs to learn how to walk and grow, and he needs to develop physically as well as emotionally. This means that you are going to need to refrain from picking him up or carrying him around with you – even if it means that you are going to have to take more time getting from one room to another. By this time in your child's life, he is going to pick things up and put them in his/her mouth more regularly.It is your job to babyproof your home and ensure there is nothing around that can cause harm to your child, and this is much better done before it becomes an issue, so make sure you take the time to do this now.

Work with your doctor to ensure that your child is on the right track when it comes to health and nutrition during this time of his life, too.

You are going to have to make sure your baby is still growing as he should, and that he is continuing to develop as he should, too. This is going to be something that your doctor can give you detailed insight on when you make your regular doctor's visits, so make sure you are open and ask any questions at all that you may have.

There is no shame at all in asking a question, especially as your child grows and changes. You want to ensure that he is getting along as he should be and know if there is anything that you can do that will aid in his growth and development.

Also, it is during the first year your child is going to start to experience separation anxiety. Again, this is something that can be worked through if you can be patient and work with your child. Use a regular caregiver when you are away so your child can become familiar with the babysitter and begin building trust.

At the same time, when it's time for you to leave, don't draw out the goodbyes – rather keep it short and sweet and head off to do what you need to do. Most children will calm down quickly, even if they were crying when you first left. If it makes you feel better, you can wait by the door to ensure that your baby does stop crying quickly, then you can carry on with your day.

1. During the first year of your child's life, you are going to start to see many of the motor skills and mental development that is going to be present in his/her toddler years, and you are going to have the chance to help them grow properly. **Things you need to do:** Babyproof your home and help your child learn how to move about the house using furniture. Make sure you turn the house into a child-friendly safety zone sooner rather than later and take the time to work with your child as he moves from space to space.

2. Work with your doctor to ensure you are on track with health and nutrition.

3. Keep goodbyes short and sweet and use the same caregiver as much as possible. The more acquainted your child becomes with the caregiver, the easier it's going to be for both of you when you are going away.

Part 2:

The Parental Survival Guide

Chapter 7

What About Me? A Parent's Guide to Sleeping

In the first part of this book, we focused our attention on how you, as the parent, are going to stand by your child every step of the way through his first year. This is something that you need to grow into and do as you are actively in the process, as there is no way you can effectively know what you are going to expect until you are right there at the moment.

At the same time, you are going to have to think about how you, as the parent, are going to continue with your real life when you have a child. Yes, when you have a baby, everything about your life is going to change, and you are going to have to do what you can to keep up with those changes. However, there are things you can do that will make this time of your life as easy as it can be, and make it so you don't hate your child's first year (as it pertains to you).

The number one complaint many new parents have is that they never get the chance to sleep. It doesn't seem to matter what they read online, they just don't find the time for themselves.

Sleep is indeed something that you are going to have to get used to doing without. But does this mean that you are going to turn into a sleep deprived monster? Not at all! During the first year of your child's life, having as much energy as possible is important, as you are also working to give your child the best start in life they can possibly have.

If there is one thing you can do that will ensure you have good sleep during your first year with your child, its teamwork. That's right – work with your partner rather than against them when it comes to sleep, and you both will find that the first year doesn't have to be as traumatizing as you feared. All too many couples choose to fight against each other when it comes to sleeping.

They both do their best to sleep through the night, then when the child begins to cry, there is a grumpy exchange as neither one want to get up and both are forced into caring for the child. This, of course, only puts strain and tension on the relationship as you are doing your best to raise your child, which is only going to lead to more stress.

The secret here is to not think about how much sleep you are getting but to look at how much sleep both of you are getting. All too often, when you are only thinking about your own schedule, neither one of you is going to get the kind of sleep that you need to be getting. So, you are going to have to work together to get through this.

And what better way to make that happen than with a schedule?

That's right, a sleep schedule. Work out with your partner the kind of sleep schedule that is going to work best for you – and stick with that. You can base this on who is working outside the home, or, if you both are, who is able to get time off and when.

You can work this out based on the day of the week, or the shift, in a sense. Decide what works for both of your schedules, be willing to compromise, and make sure the both of you are getting the rest you need. When you are both willing to work together on the sleeping, you are going to find that while neither one of you are going to get the full amount of sleep that you want to get, you are going to get enough to make it work well for the both of you.

This is going to take time and practice, and it's going to require that you are both willing to work together to find something that works for both of you. The more you are willing to compromise for the good of your partner, the more you are going to find something that meets in the middle, and the better you're going to feel when it comes to taking care of your child.

All too many people feel that during the first year, they are only going to be taking care of the baby, and as a result, they tend to do things that end up hurting the entire situation in the long run. Make sure you are working together to raise your child, and you are going to find that the task isn't as hard as you think it's going to be.

There is no wrong way to work together, as long as you are both making the compromises and sacrifices to make sure both of you are happy with the results at the end of the day. It's going to be worth it.

From the moment your child is born, you are going to:

1. Work with your partner to ensure both of you are getting the sleep that you need. Don't be worried about just your own sleep, worry about your partner's as well.

2. Set up a sleep schedule for you and your partner as well as for the baby. This will help ensure that you and your partner, including your baby, get the proper amount of sleep that you need.

3. Compromise. The more you are willing to work together, the better it is going to be for the both of you – and for the baby as well.

Chapter 8:

Yours, Mine, and Ours: Connecting as Parents

If you were to ask any parent, "What is one of the largest strains on a marriage?" you are going to hear that children add a lot more stress than they ever thought they would. One always think that once the kids come along, everything is going to be just fine for the parents. They are going to work together, the children are always going to be quiet and happy, and everything is going to suddenly morph into a happy family of perfection that no one ever thinks anything negative about.

However, the reality is babies put all kinds of stress and tension on a relationship, and this is largely going to make it harder for you to do many of the things that you once did. When you were used to going out and connecting as a couple before, you are going to find that you have to stay in and take care of the baby. When you were able to go on vacations and not worry about the cost before, you are going to find that now there are more bills than you know what to do with.

Sure, there is going to be another little child in the mix that you love more than anything, but when it comes down to you and your partner, you are going to find that the one thing that draws you both together is also the one thing that drives you apart.

It is only natural that parents find peace and joy in solitude, meaning there is going to be a lot less time for you and your partner getting it on in the bathroom or in the closet like you used to do. Now, you are going to find that there is such joy in being alone, the both of you are more likely going to seek that out rather than being with each other.

Although when you read this for the first time, it does sound rather bleak, but it doesn't need to be this way. As with the subject of sleeping that we looked at in the last chapter, if you are willing to work with your partner on this issue, you are going to find that you are able to get through this without any problems, too.

When it comes to raising your child, the best thing you can do to stay connected with your partner is to work together with your partner to ensure that you are both doing the right thing. You need to support your partner during this time, and you need to be in agreement on the direction that you wish to move in with your child.

This is a truth that is going to last no matter how old the child is, and it is something that is going to keep your marriage strong throughout the years. Yes, there is going to be a strain on the relationship from time to time, and there are going to be things that you do and don't agree on, but when it comes down to the core values of you and your partner, you need to make sure you are on the same page.

Before your baby is born, sit down with your partner and work out the finer details of what you want to do with your child. These are things such as the style of parenting you are going to have – how are you going to teach your child sign language?

When are you going to take time for yourselves? How are you going to sleep? What are you going to do with the baby when it comes to such things as work and the other obligations of life?

When there are so many questions that need to be addressed, it is far better to work with your partner from the beginning. Know what to expect and make sure they do as well. There is no wrong way to love your child, but there is a way you can do it that is going to bring you and your partner together. When you know that there is trust between the two of you, and you are both working together for the common goal, then you are going to be better able to work together when it comes to the little things in your relationship.

As with the sleeping, you are going to have to find the compromise that works for both you and your partner. Instead of being forceful and doing what you think you are supposed to do, act out of love and support for your partner. Be understanding of the stress and hardship that is placed on them throughout all of this, and see how you can work together to make it easier on both of you.

The more you are able to work on things with the common goal at the end, the better you are going to find this transition goes. You are going to stay together throughout all of this, so work together on it from the beginning.

You are each other's strongest ally in all of this, so act like it, and conquer what life is throwing your way.

1. **What you need to do:** Put your partner first when you are thinking of doing anything. Ask yourself if there is anything you can do that will make your partner feel loved and valued, and see if there is a way you can make this transition easier on your partner. If you are both doing this, you are going to be amazed at how easy the change is.

2. Don't worry about how even the division is. If you are both thinking of the other person, you are going to find that no one person is stuck with doing everything.

3. Focus on how you can grow as a couple as you become parents. This is something that you are both going to have to learn how to do, and it is something that is

going to come with time. When neither one of you know how to do something, it is the perfect opportunity to learn together.

4. Be each other's greatest support system. Nothing is going to shake you when you know that you can turn to your partner for support and love, and they can do the same with you!

Chapter 9

Two's Company: Co-Parenting the Right Way

In the last chapter, we looked at ways you can connect with your partner when it comes to raising your child. Now, this is something that is a little different than co-parenting, though the two are closely tied.

When it comes to connecting with your partner, you are going to focus on doing things that build your partner and the relationship up. These are things that are going to bring the two of you together as much as possible. When it comes to co-parenting, you are going to be focused on raising your child together, as partners.

Your child is going to look to both of you when it comes to growing, and they are going to need both of you to be an active part in their lives. This is going to be something that you are going to work out with your partner from the beginning, but it is also going to take daily discipline to ensure that you are really going to go through with it.

It is easier said than done, to be sure, but co-parenting is something that is foundational in any family, no matter what the other circumstances are.

As we mentioned before in the last chapter, this is something that you are going to work out with your partner before the baby arrives. As difficult as it is, you need to know in advance the big things before the moment arrives. This is going to make it easier to go through with the transition when you have to live it.

You know how you were raised, and from that, you know the things that you want to do and the things that you don't want to do. You know what is important, the things that weren't really a big deal when you were a kid, and the things that aren't really a big deal to you now. When it comes to raising your own child, you are going to want to discuss these things with your partner before you even begin.

Think about such things as spiritual beliefs, how you are going to handle extended family, and what you are going to do when it comes to such things as discipline, family life, and other things that affect your child as well as the both of you. Think of the general ways you want your family to be run and work out with your partner how you are going to accomplish this.

Although two people are able to live together without too many troubles with certain things when they are individuals, this changes when there is a baby in the mix. You are going to have to suddenly think about how your decisions are going to affect your child and what you can do that will make this a harmonic place for all of you.

You don't want there to be any tension in the years to come, and this is all going to begin when your baby is on the way. How are you going to handle the questions from the nosy Aunt Polly? What are you going to do about the baptism? How are you going to raise your child in the holidays?

There are so many things you need to take into account, and these are things that are going to only grow as time passes. Sure, you might not have to worry about them at first, but as your child grows and develops into their own person, you will have to worry about it more and more, and it is something that you are going to have to take into consideration in the years to come.

With this in mind, don't worry about putting it off, instead, address these issues in the beginning. Don't let there be any secrets between you and your partner, and don't let things that are going to be big deals just go by the wayside. At the same time, it is important for the two of you to compromise and find ways that will work for the both of you. It isn't fair for one of you to expect your child to be raised a certain way when the other one is set against it – look for a way to meet in the middle.

Parenthood is one of the most difficult things you will experience in your life, but when you are preparing for it, you can do things with your partner that is going to make life a lot easier. The more you are able to work with your partner, the more you realize you are not alone in this, and the better you will be able to face the changes that are coming your way.

What you need to do before the baby arrives:

1. Work out your parenting style with your partner – discuss the things that are important to you and how you are going to accomplish them in your family life.

2. Work out how you are going to continue to be partners in this new transition. There are so many unknowns and working together with your partner, being on the same page on many of the things that you weren't before is important.

3. Don't be afraid to work out the hard things before you move on to the next. You are going to be far happier knowing that you are on the same page than if you are working against each other with your baby in the middle.

4. Remember that this is a work in progress and you learn as you go, with each of you willing to compromise on some things.

Chapter 10

Party of One: The Art of Alone Time

While there is so much to be said for a family that is constantly together, there is also a lot to be said for spending time alone. When you become a parent, you are going to find that your alone time is virtually non-existent, and you will have to learn how to function without it.

Though many people think that they won't ever want to be alone again when they first lay their eyes on their child, but this is something that must be understood because everyone needs a few minutes to themselves each day, and it is important that you are still getting yours. **When it comes to parenthood, scheduling your alone time is as important as scheduling everything else in your life.** You might begin to feel as though you are a slave to your schedule, but the fact of the matter is that you aren't. You want to still be in control of your life, and if you are going to do this, you must know what to expect. When it comes to a newborn child or even a child that is a few months old to even a year old, you are going to spend so much time chasing them around and doing what they are doing that you aren't going to have the time to yourself anymore.

This means that if you still want to do certain things in your life, you must schedule them – that's right, on pen and paper.

Don't be afraid to pen into the mix the fact that you are going to be spending time alone, and make sure that you take this time to truly do things that you enjoy. This could be something as simple as taking a hot bath and letting the day soak away into the tub, or it might be taking a class or going out and pampering yourself.

Make sure you discuss with your partner ways you are going to spend time to yourselves while you raise your child, and also work together to ensure the two of you really get this time to yourselves. Don't be afraid to tell your partner that you are going to go do something, and you are going to need them to watch your child for a while. Make sure this is something that works for your partner and be willing to compromise with them. If you are able to always swap out the time you spend alone, as well as make time for both of you to spend time together, you are going to find that the time that you spend in the stressful situations of parenting is much easier to handle.

When parenting is stressful, most parents don't realize they truly just need to take a few minutes to themselves. They end up forcing themselves to continue to work through it, without ever taking a breather. Though this might seem like the noble thing to do, it ends up causing strain all around.

Be willing to take time for yourself. You both need it.

During the first year (and into the later years of parenting) you will:

1. Discuss with your partner on how you are both going to get your own time in the mix of things. Be willing to compromise to ensure that both of you are getting your time alone.

2. Work together to be alone. Take the time to just have a few minutes to yourself at the end of the day (or first thing in the morning).

3. Don't be afraid to voice your needs, but at the same time, be willing to work with your partner to ensure that it works for everyone.

Part 3:

Tell Me What You Really Think: Baby Sign Language

Chapter 11:

Baby Sign Language: Everything You Need to Know

One of the biggest sources of stress new parents face is the fact that they aren't sure of what to do when their child is needing something. So often, a new parent will say that they just wish their child is able to talk to them and tell them what they need – but they are too little to speak.

This only results in frustration for both parents as well as the child, and it is something that every new parent dreads. However, it doesn't need to be this way, and with the proper technique, you can teach your child how to interact with you in a way that you can understand from a very young age.

I am referring to baby sign language.

That's right. Babies who are only a few months old can learn the art of sign language, and as a result, they are going to be able to tell you exactly what they want and when they want it.

This, as you can imagine, is going to remove a lot of the stress you feel as a parent, and it is going to put you back in control when it comes to knowing what your baby needs. After all, wouldn't you like to simply ask your baby what they want at any given moment and have them tell you directly what they are feeling? This is going to make it far easier for you as the parent to provide for them in the exact way that they need, and it is also going to remove the stress from you.

Now, to teach your baby sign language, it's going to require that you do two things:

1. You are going to have to learn the art of sign language yourself and

2. You are going to have to teach your child how to do it.

Thankfully, when it comes to baby sign language, you are not alone. There are literally hundreds of resources online that are all going to show you exactly what you need to do when it comes to teaching your child sign language, with detailed lessons and practices that you can work on both by yourself and with your child. And in no time at all, you will find that he is able to tell you exactly what you want – and you can do the same.

Baby sign language can be as in depth or as basic as you want it to be, as long as you are able to understand what it is your child is saying. You don't have to be completely fluent in sign language yourself, in fact, it is often better if you are going to learn with your baby – and with your partner as well. If you would like, you can both learn something that is only specific to your own family – make up your own language, which you are all able to understand.

If on the other hand you want to go with something that is more conventional, you can do with the standard way of learning, which means you are going to use such things as the internet and YouTube. Simply get online and search for how to teach your child sign language and begin the lessons. You can decide when you want your child to begin learning and you can cater to that in your own lessons, or you can go with it if your child is already a bit older.

When it comes to teaching your child sign language, you really are in control of how and when your child learns. Just learn to work with your child and with your partner in the direction you are going and you are going to find that the transition is easy and smooth.

Practice makes perfect.

Babies as young as six months old can learn sign language, and it has been suggested that babies even younger can learn some of the most basic signs.

When it comes to communication with your baby, the more basic you can go, the better. Instead of going with full sentences or trying to have a conversation with your child, simply go with the most simple of communication.

Teach your child how to tell you what he wants and only what he wants. There's no need to go beyond that. At the same time, teach your child how to say please and thank you, and make sure you do the same when you are talking to them. When it comes to communication with your child, remember that consistency is the best thing you can do.

Think of it as teaching your child how to literally converse with you and you aren't going to have any issues at all discussing with them what you want them to do. Just as you work with your child when you talk about such things as mama and dada, you are going to do the same with your words in the signed realm.

Again, if you sign on to various sources online, you will find that there are all sorts of ways you can work with your child from the beginning. You will see that the more you work with them, the faster they are going to pick up on what you are teaching them and the more they are going to branch out and learn the new words you want them to know.

Treat your child as though you are already having a conversation with them and you will see that they will soon pick up on the communication that you're using with them. When you get your partner on board with this concept, you are going to find that this process happens even faster. The key is to be consistent and work with your child.

Reward your child as you go along and show them that you are responding to what it is they are saying. The more they get results from what they are telling you, the easier it is going to be for them to understand what you are saying when you communicate with them. As with every other aspect of parenthood, this is something you pick up and learn over time.

Get your partner on board from the beginning and the two of you are going to find that this is one of the easiest, fastest, and most stress-reducing ways you can communicate with your child.

Give yourself time and work with your child as well as with yourself. You will find that this isn't as hard as you think it's going to be, and in no time at all, you are going to become the type of parent you have always wanted to be.

Chapter 12:

Signs of The Times: Teaching Your Child Sign Language

The first year of your baby is the first step to a long life, and communication is vital to a happy family life. Babies are ready for their parents to start signing to them after four months old. However, they will sign back after nine months. I aim to help your baby learn the first 10 basic signs that your baby will use frequently (nad likely every day) for better communication. As your baby signs back to you, your communication will be better.

Teaching Baby Signs :

These are the three principles that will help you teach your baby sign language:

- **Fun**- Sign playfully and make a game out of it – motivation to learn is key!

- **Repetition**- Repetition is always essential for better communication. Pracitce daily to help your baby learn quickly.

- **Encourage**- Progress should be rewarded with praise and attention.

Here are the **<u>10 basic and most common signs</u>** to help your baby express himself/ herself .

- ✓ Mom, Mother, Mommy
- ✓ Dad, Father, Daddy
- ✓ Eat/ Food
- ✓ Milk
- ✓ Dog
- ✓ Cat
- ✓ More
- ✓ All Done
- ✓ Bath
- ✓ Sleep

Please note that these are basic baby signs. There will be more baby signs and they will be described better in the second edition of this book.

Mom, Mother, Mommy

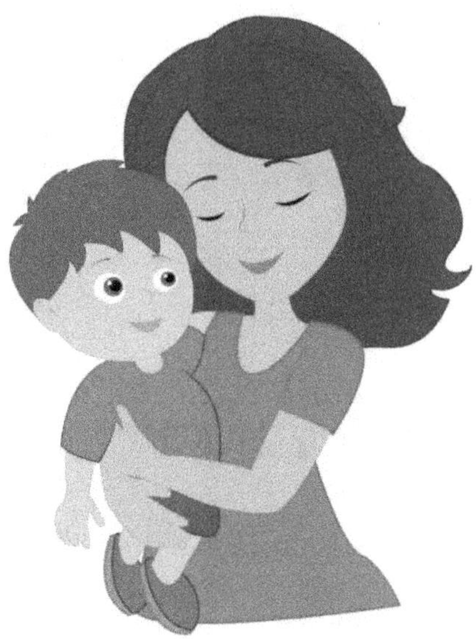

To sign mommy
extend and spread
your fingers apart.
With your pinkie
facing forward tap
your thumb on your
chin.

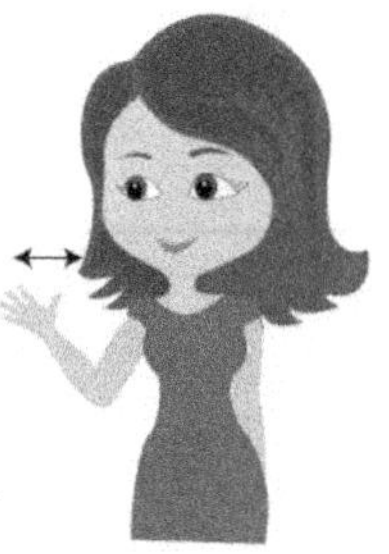

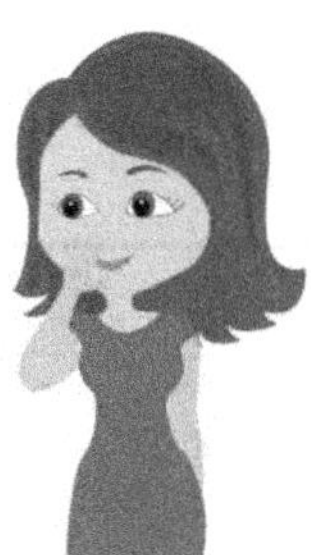

Father ,Dad, Daddy

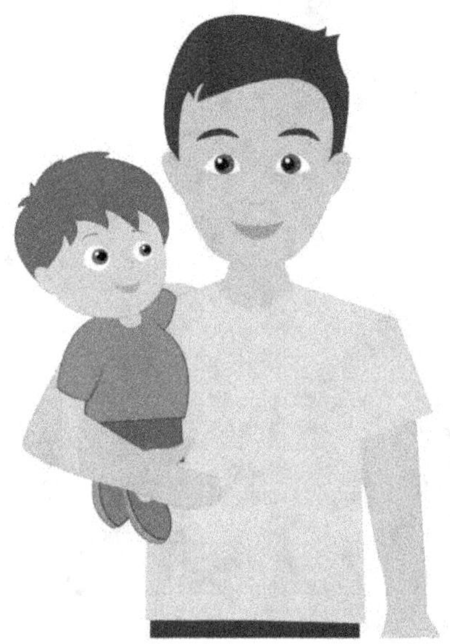

To sign daddy, extend and spread out your five fingers on your strong hand. Tap your hand on your forehead.

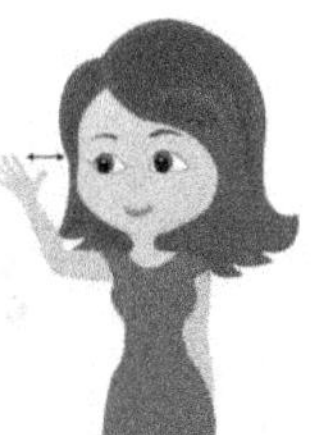

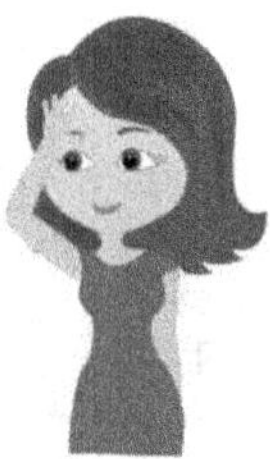

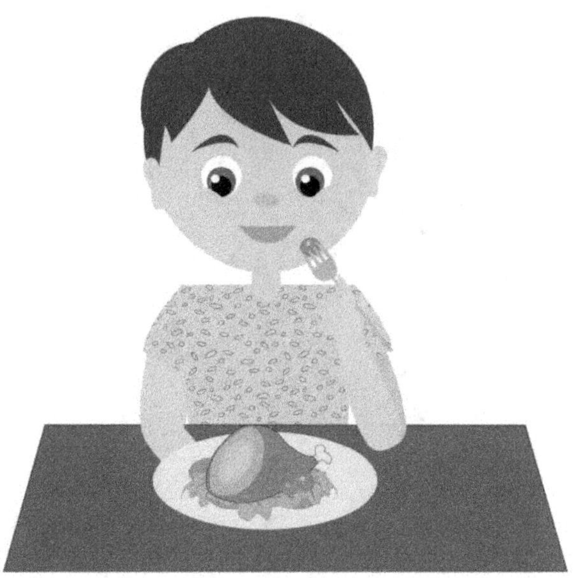

 Make the sign for eat by taking you strong hand, with the tip of your thumb touching the tips of your fingers and tapping it on your mouth. (The universal sign for eating) The same sign is used for food.

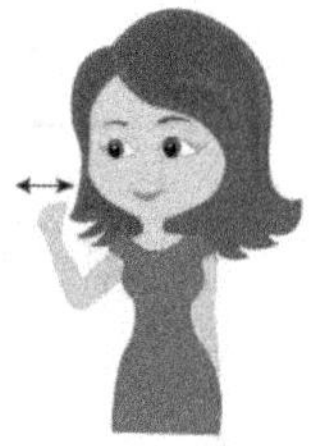

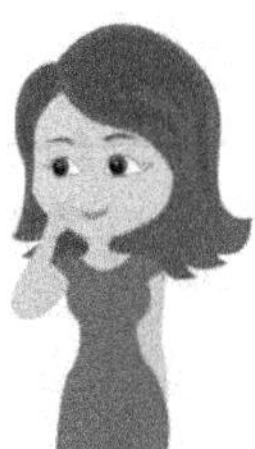

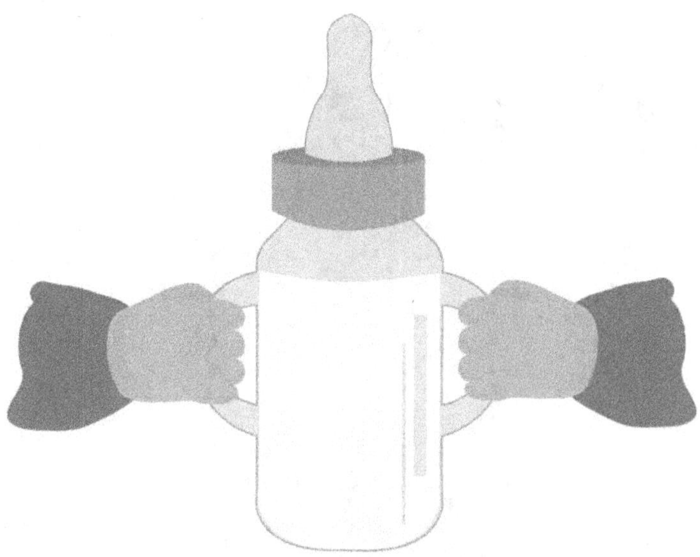

The milk sign is a lot like milking a cow (or goat), but without the vertical motion – you are just squeezing the udder. You take both hands, make them into a fist, relax, and repeat.

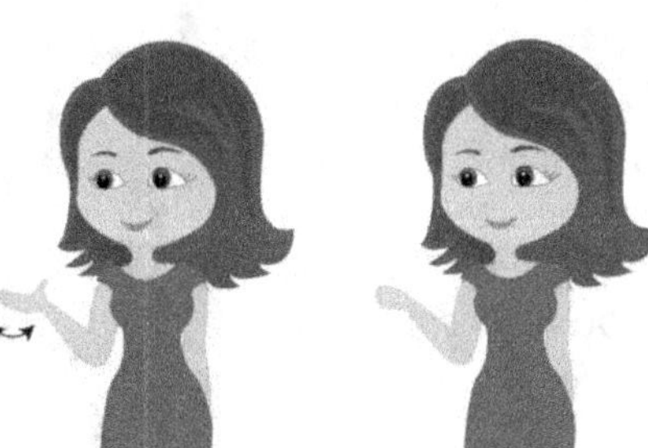

Dog

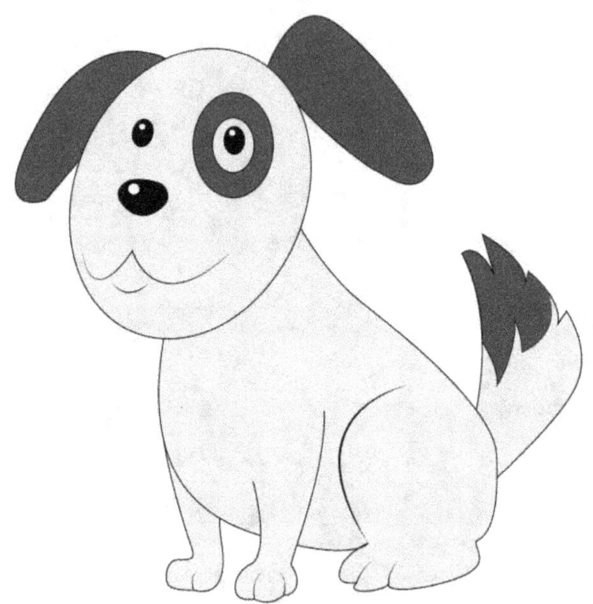

Sign dog by patting your outstretched hand with fingers together on the side of your hip. Just as if you were calling the dog.

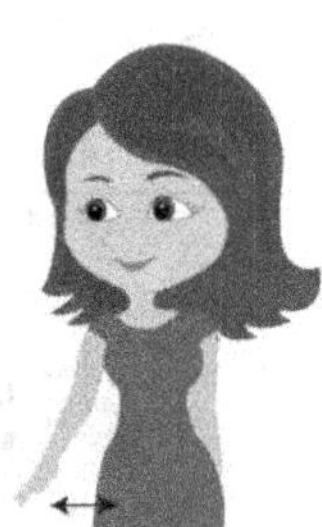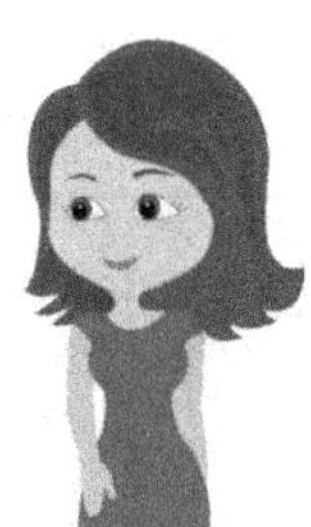

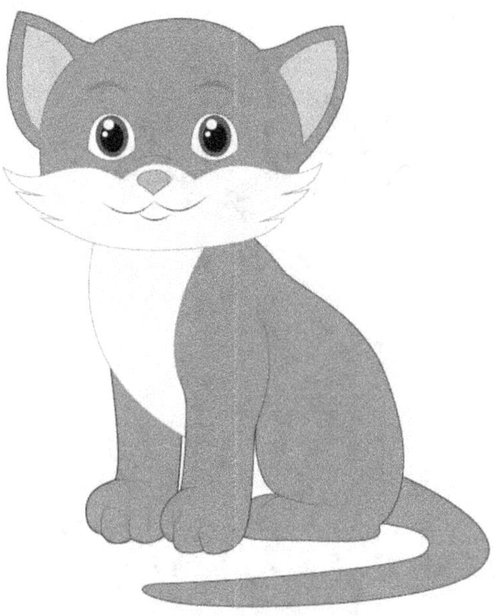

To sign cat, with both hands pinch your thumb and index finger together by the side of each cheek, while keeping your remaining fingers straight out. As you pinch your fingers together take them from each side of your face outward. The sign looks just like you are teasing your whiskers straight.

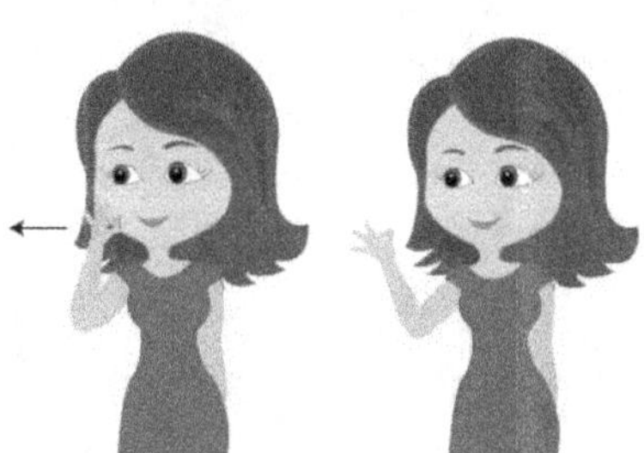

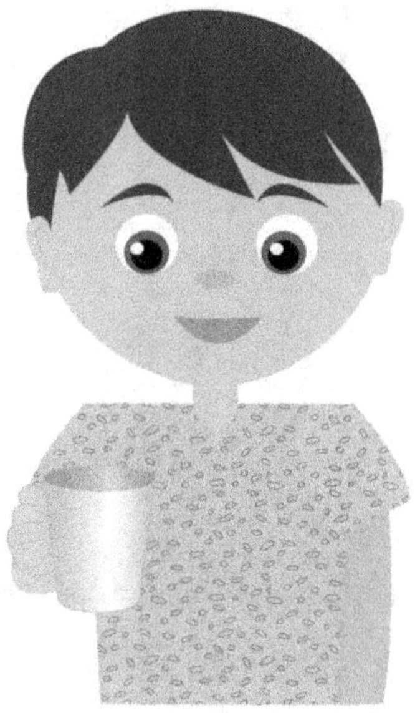

To do the sign for more, flatten out your hands then bring your thumbs under to make an O shape. Then, bring your hands together and separate them repeatedly.

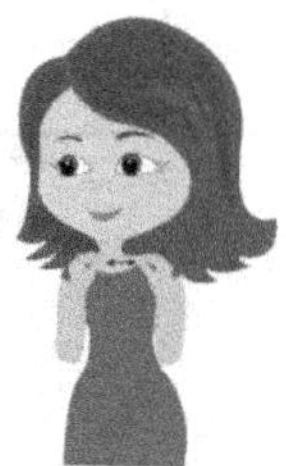 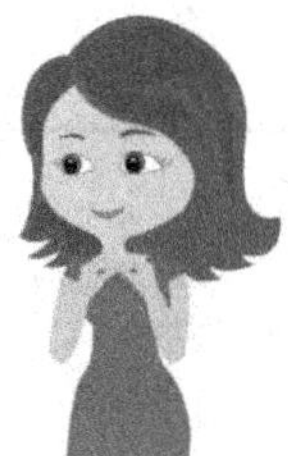

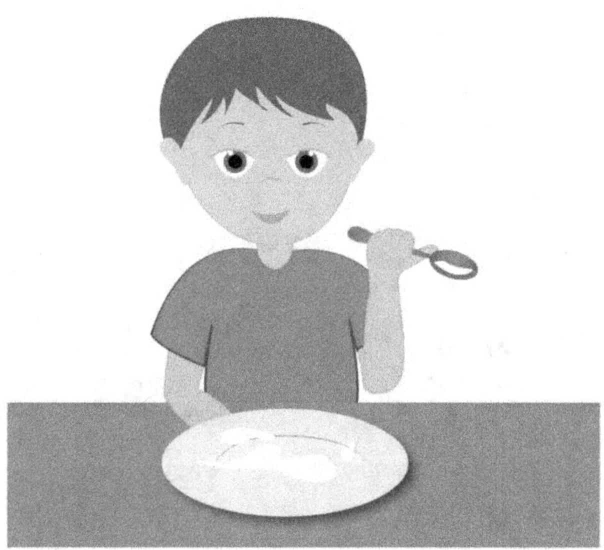

The sign for finished, looks like you are pushing something away with your pinkies. Start the sign by taking both your hands opened up and palms facing you. Flick your hands round so that you end with your palms facing out.

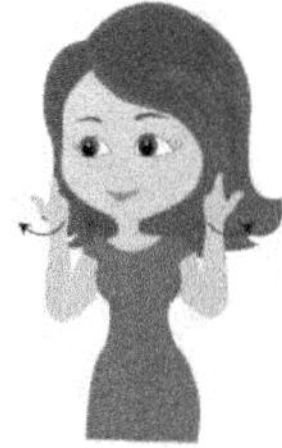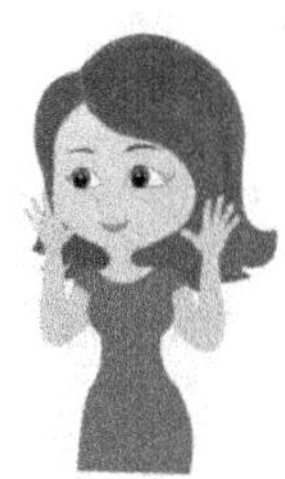

BATH

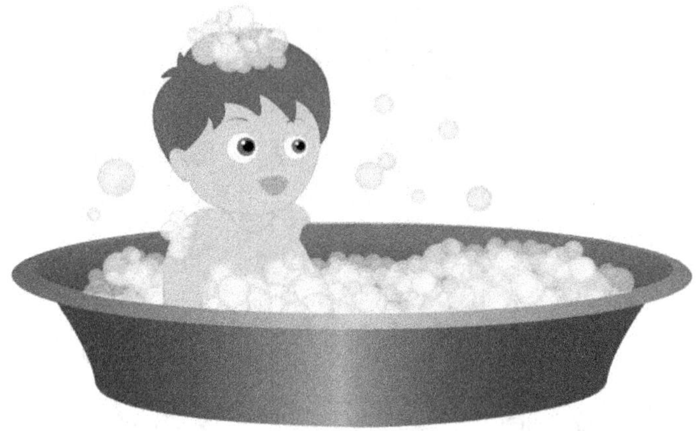

 Sign bath, by making a fist out of your two hands, then moving the fists vertically up and down your chest. The sign looks a lot like someone scrubbing themselves with both hands, as if taking a very efficient bath

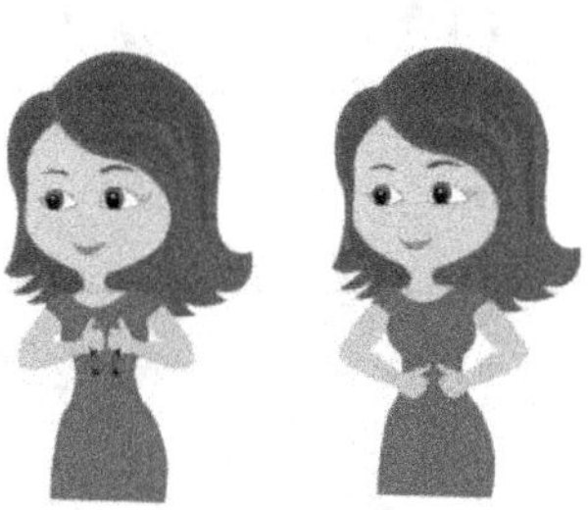

SLEEP

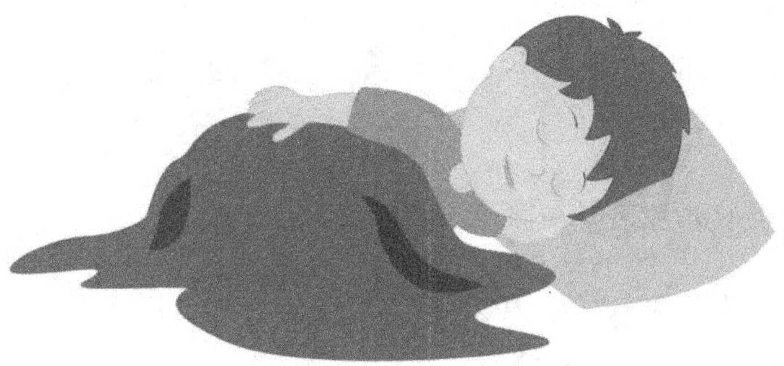

To sign sleep, start with fingers extended and spread apart. Beginning with your hand over your face, move your fingers down to end with your hand below your chin and your fingers touching your thumb. As you make the sign, feel your face relax and your eyes get droopy to add to the sleepy effect.

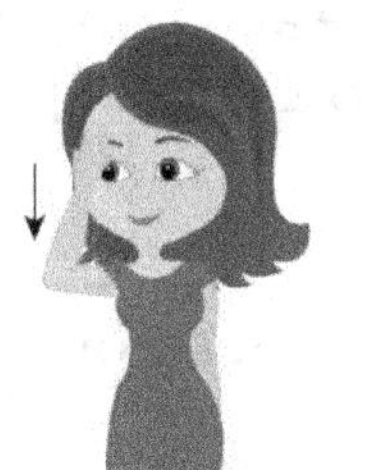
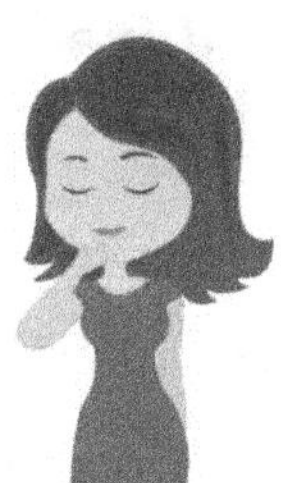

....

Before we wrap up this book, I do have one favor to ask of you. Please take a minute and write an honest review on the Amazon page.

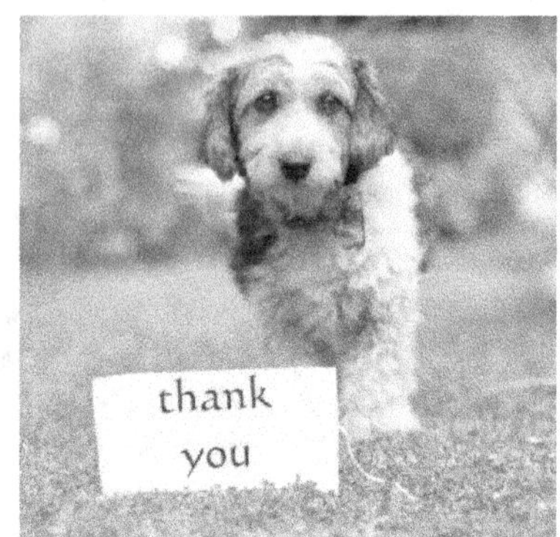

Reviews are the lifeblood of our books and I would greatly appreciate your thoughts on it!

Please go to amazon.com and search with book title and leave an honest review.

Your Baby's First Year : Enjoying Your Baby's First Year With Baby Sign Language

Or

Please check-it-out the link below.

http://amzn.to/2oHgUsG

....

Thanks ! Now, continue on the next page.

Conclusion

There you have it, everything you need to know to survive and enjoy the first year of your child's life. I hope this book was able to show you that you really can take charge of this year, and you can live through each of the stages, offering your child everything there is to offer while you still get the time to take care of yourself.

I hope you found this book inspiring and you take what you have learned here and apply it to your life and your situation. Let this book erase the fear you may feel during this time and give you the confidence in its place.

Your child deserves nothing but the best and you can give them the very best. All it takes is some confidence that you are doing the right thing and you'll see that you can approach this year like a boss.

Parenting is the most important thing you will ever do in your life, so ***let's make it the best first year ever!***

You'll want to do it again.

Thank you and Good luck!

Nicole Johnson

BONUS!

Wouldn't be nice to discover and learn sleep tips for babies in a such way that you would sleep while your angel sleep well. Well now is your chance!

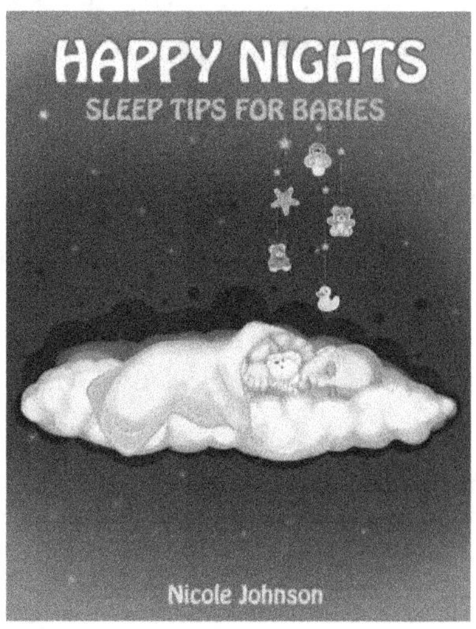

Please check it out   http://bit.ly/2BXvkaZ

Simply as a 'Thank you' for downloading this book, I would like to give you full access to an exclusive that will email you notifications when Amazon's top Kindle Books go on Free Promotion. If you are someone who is interested in saving a ton of money, then simply click the link for FREE access.